Mediterranean Diet

A Simple Cookbook & Guide For Busy People To Rapid Weight Loss & Healthy Eating Mastery

Table of Contents

Introduction

I want to thank you and congratulate you for buying the book "Mediterranean Diet: A Simple Cookbook & Guide For Busy People To Rapid Weight Loss And Healthy Eating Mastery"

The Mediterranean tradition offers a cuisine rich in colors, aromas and memories, which support the taste and the spirit of those who live in harmony with nature. Everyone is talking about the Mediterranean diet, but few are those who do it properly, thus generating a lot of confusion for the reader. And so some associate it with pizza, others identify it with noodles combined with meat sauce, in a mixture of pseudo historical traditions and folklore that do not help to solve the question that is at the basis of any diet: combining and balancing the food so as to satisfy the qualitative and quantitative needs of an individual and in a sense, preserving their health through the use of substances that help the body to perform normal vital functions.

Mastering the Mediterranean Diet

Where It All Began

The varied cuisines of the Mediterranean have developed over the millennia, with notable regional changes happening with the introduction of New World foods starting in the 16th century. The concept of a Mediterranean cuisine, however, is very recent. Although it was first publicized in 1945 by the American doctor Ancel Keys stationed in Salerno, Italy, the Mediterranean diet failed to gain widespread recognition until the 1990s. Our collective obsession with the Mediterranean diet and lifestyle began in the late 1950s when scientists noticed that Spain, Italy, Southern France, Greece and Turkey experienced far fewer deaths from heart disease than most other countries in the world. They eventually determined that low intakes of saturated fat were one of the diet's features that protected the hearts of people in the region. Objective data showing that the Mediterranean diet is healthy, first originated from the Seven Countries Study. The Mediterranean diet is based on what from the point of view of mainstream nutrition is considered a paradox: that although the people living in Mediterranean countries tend to consume relatively high amounts of fat, they have far lower rates of cardiovascular disease than in countries like the United States, where similar levels of fat consumption arefound.

A number of diets have received attention, but the strongest evidence for a beneficial health effect and decreased mortality after switching to a largely plant based diet comes from studies of Mediterranean diet, e.g. from the NIH-AARP Diet and Health Study. The Mediterranean diet is often cited as beneficial for being low in saturated fat and high in monounsaturated fat and dietary fiber. One of the main explanations is thought to be the health effects of olive oil included in the Mediterranean diet. The Mediterranean diet is high in salt content.Foods such as olives, salt-cured cheeses, anchovies, capers, salted fish roe, and salads dressed with extra virgin olive oil all contain high levels of salt. The inclusion of red wine is considered a factor contributing to health as it contains flavonoids with powerful antioxidant properties.

The Science Behind The Mediterranean Diet

Although the Mediterranean diet is traditionally low in saturated fat, it is by no means a low-fat diet. The typical diet is made up of large amounts of healthy fats from nuts, fish and vegetable oils; an abundance of vegetables, fruits and legumes; and whole grain breads and cereals. Healthy fats like mono- and polyunsaturates have several health benefits. For one, they lower blood cholesterol levels. Research spanning several decades suggests that healthy fats may also promote heart health by preventing the formation of blood clots in our arteries and preventing abnormal heart rhythms. And the benefits of the healthy fats, vegetables, fruit and whole grains in traditional Mediterranean diets extend beyond heart health. A 2008 study of more than 380,000 American men and women found that those who followed the Mediterranean-style diet closely, versus those who did not, had a 20% reduced risk of death from any cause.

Benefits Of The Diet

Here's what science has to say about the positive effects of the eating habits of Mediterranean natives:

Keeps elders agile:

A 2012 study conducted on elderly residents of Tuscany, Italy, found that keeping to a Mediterranean-style diet decreased a senior's odds of developing hallmark signs of frailty (slow walking speed, muscle weakness, generalized exhaustion) by about 70 percent, when compared to those who subscribed to a different nutritional program. Avoiding signs of frailty can help prevent falls, fractures and broken bones in the elderly.

Fights chronic ailments:

Study after study shows how Mediterranean diet foods can help reduce a person's risk for developing chronic illnesses, including heart disease, diabetes, cancer, arthritis, dental disease, macular degeneration and Alzheimer's. They may also play a role in helping people with asthma and chronic obstructive pulmonary disease (COPD) manage their condition.

Protects the brain:

Adhering to healthy lifestyle practices may reduce a person's risk of Alzheimer's disease and other cognitive disorders. Dietary habits can and do have profound effects on our brains both directly, as well as indirectly. A good diet is one that is high in fruits, vegetables and whole grains, and low in dairy, saturated fat and refined sugar (a.k.a. the Mediterranean diet). The positive effects on memory function associated with a brain-healthy diet may be as effective (or even more effective over time) than those achieved with current FDA-approved medications.

The Mediterranean Diet test

Tricks And Tips

1. Eat more fruit and salad

Make sure you eat fruit and veg at every meal and choose them as snacks and puddings too. Make a green salad more interesting by introducing tomatoes and peppers, and fruits such as figs, pomegranates, citrus fruits and grapes.

2. Have meat-free days

The Mediterranean diet typically includes more fish and less meat. Going for fish, beans and pulses is a good way to increase your protein.

3. Focus on 'good' fats

Unsaturated fats are the main type of fat used in the Mediterranean, most famously olive oil. Replace butter, lard and ghee with unsaturated oils from plants and seeds such as olive and rapeseed oil. This can help to lower your cholesterol levels.

4. Make it your own

Mediterranean flavours may not lend themselves to all cuisines, but that doesn't mean you still can't adopt some of the elements of this approach. For example, if you are cooking a spicy dish such as curry and you're looking for a healthier alternative to ghee, use coconut or palm oil.

5. Drink sensibly

Many people assume that wine is a key element of the Mediterranean diet, but it is optional. If you do drink, it's important to keep it in moderation.

6. Make sure half your plate is covered with different colored vegetables.

When you tell people to eat vegetables, they often think they have to make a special trip to a farmer's market and then clean the vegetables, which can become a burden. But good vegetables can be found in the freezer section of the supermarket. Nutrients are really packed in when the freezing plant is close to the farm, and that's better than 'fresh' vegetables that have been sitting in a warehouse for a month.

7. Use unsaturated oils such as olive oil or canola.

Extra virgin olive oil is rich in polyphenols, which come from the skin of the olive. Polyphenols have been shown to be beneficial to heart health.

8. Don't fall for the "100% wheat" gimmick on bread labels.

Whole grains are important because when you eat whole grain, you get anti-oxidants as well as fiber. But some bread labels are misleading. If the first ingredient doesn't have the word 'whole' in it, such as 'whole wheat flour,' it's not whole grain.

Dining the Mediterranean way

The Mediterranean Beginner's plate

The traditional Mediterranean lifestyle emphasizes the importance of people eating healthfully together among family and friends. The act of cooking, eating, and cleaning up a meal is something that is done with others.

Between demanding jobs and busy personal schedules, many of us have gotten away from sitting down together at the kitchen table.

Try to make a conscious effort to slow down your pace and get your family involved in the kitchen:

- Pick out healthy recipes together to try.

- Buy healthy foods together at your local farmer's market or grocery store.

- Cook them together in the kitchen.

- Sit down as a family to enjoy a meal together.

Not only will this contribute to your physical health, but it can do wonders for your emotional and mental health as well.

The Mediterranean guide to eating and shopping

The Mediterranean Diet is about day to day simple patterns of eating and ingredients rather than complex cuisine or time consuming recipes, unless of course there is special occasion to celebrate. Referring to the Mediterranean Diet Pyramid, a visit to the supermarket can ensure stocks of basic ingredients easily accessible to create a wonderful food experience. Brown rice, pasta, couscous, other whole grains and potatoes can form the low GI carbohydrate which combine with vegetables or beans and perhaps fish, lean white or red meat to create a balanced , nutritious and complete meal.

Salads are a beautiful accompaniment to fish and meat, in particular combining the colours of a summer garden at any time of year. Herbs and spices are readily available in packets, dried or fresh to add flavour and variety to meals. They can even be purchased in convenient plastic tubes. Alternatively potted herbs around the kitchen or patio, replaced from time to time, allows fresh leaves to be always available.

"Jazzing up the Carb"

The lowly potato, so common in Western European diets can be given the "Positively Good for You" Mediterranean treatment. Try baked potatoes seared with fresh rosemary and a little garlic, or part boiled and sliced potatoes roasted until crisp with a drizzle of olive oil and a sprinkle of paprika. Why not pour a little passata over the roasting vegetables and throw some basil leaves on at the time of serving? And what about "mash with a dash" – mashed potato with a dash of olive oil and crushed garlic or chilli!

Similarly brown rice is wholesome simply boiled but can add flavour and goodness to a meal with fried or raw red or spring onion and herbs sprinkled on top. Perhaps fry the onion in a little ginger from a bottle or tube.

Salads – endless combinations

At least once try the "super- salad" loaded with antioxidants and colour; the only challenge will be finding a bowl big enough! This can be served with grilled lean meat or fish and olive oil roasted potatoes.

Include: lettuce, tomatoes, pitted olives, mixed nuts, red onion, beetroot, radish, mixed peppers, sun dried tomatoes, finely chopped carrots, fresh bay leaves, cucumber, red grapes, seeds and a sprinkle of grated cheese or feta. Perhaps add a little avocado...

Dressings, instant marinades, and drizzles

To accompany a salad, to drizzle onto vegetables or to marinate or glaze grilled roast meat and fish, simply mix up a special olive oil dressing. Again the combination of flavours from simple and positively good for you ingredients is almost endless.

From a basic mix of extra virgin olive oil with balsamic vinegar or walnut oil, the scope for dressings is wide and can include many ingredients which combine healthy antioxidants with fabulous flavours. A dressing might include olive oil, perhaps combined with some flax oil and lemon juice, sundried tomato paste, honey, chopped garlic and herbs. Some chopped chilli or mustard will add spice and white wine or balsamic vinegar can enhance the rich "peppery" experience.

If used as a glaze, a little yoghurt can be placed lightly on top of the meat. The spice route passed through the Mediterranean and the spice markets of Istanbul combined traditional herbs of the Mediterranean with more exotic flavours from India and the Far East. Stir frying vegetables with seafood or meats in olive oil with spices such as chilli, turmeric, ginger and soy sauce is a great way to include such produce.

Mediterranean Recipes

Mediterranean Salad Recipes

Potato Salad

Total time: 24 minutes

Prep time: 10 minutes

Cook time: 14 minutes

Yield: 4 servings

Ingredients Potato

- 5 medium potatoes, peeled and diced

- Coarse salt, to taste

- ¼ onion

- 3 tbsp. yellow mustard

- 2 cups mayonnaise

- 1 tsp. paprika, sweet

- 1 tsp. Tabasco

- 2 scallions, thinly sliced

Directions

- Pour some water in a saucepan and place over medium heat.

- Add the potatoes, season with coarse salt and boil for around 10 minutes until tender.

- Drain the water and return the saucepan to the heat to dry them out.

- Let the potatoes cool to room temperature.

- Grate the onion in a mixing bowl, add mustard, mayo, paprika and the hot sauce and mix well.

- Add the potatoes to the bowl and toss until evenly coated.

- Divide among four bowls and top with the sliced scallions.

Italian Bread Salad

Total time: 2 hours 30 minutes

Prep time: 25 minutes, plus 2 hours Refrigerator time

Cook time: 5 minutes

Yield: 4 servings

Ingredients

- 3 tbsp. freshly squeezed lemon juice

- 2 tbsp. extra virgin olive oil

- Sea salt

- Freshly ground pepper

- 1 red onion, halved and sliced

- 1 bulb fennel, stalks removed and sliced

- 1 peeled English cucumber, sliced

- 1 ½ pounds diced tomatoes

- ⅓ cup pitted Kalamata olives, halved

- 4 slices whole-wheat country bread

- 1 garlic clove, peeled and halved

- 4 ounces shaved ricotta salata cheese

- ½ cup fresh basil leaves

Directions

- Whisk together lemon juice and extra virgin olive oil in a large bowl; season with sea salt and black pepper.

- Stir in onion, fennel, cucumber, tomatoes, and olives; toss to combine and refrigerate for about 2 hours.

- When ready, heat your broiler with the rack positioned 4 inches from heat and toast the bread on a baking sheet for about 2 minutes per side or until lightly browned.

- Transfer the toasted bread to a work surface and rub with the cut garlic and cut it into 2-inch pieces.

- Divide the bread among four shallow bowls and top with the tomato salad; sprinkle with cheese and basil to serve.

Mediterranean Quinoa Salad

Total time: 35 minutes

Prep time: 15 minutes

Cook time: 20 minutes

Yield: 4 servings

Ingredients

- 1 clove garlic, smashed
- 2 cups water
- 2 cubes chicken bouillon
- 1 cup uncooked quinoa
- ½ cup chopped Kalamata olives
- 1 large red onion, diced
- 2 large chicken breasts (cooked), diced
- 1 large green bell pepper, diced
- ½ cup crumbled feta cheese
- ¼ cup chopped fresh chives
- ¼ cup chopped fresh parsley
- ½ tsp. sea salt
- ¼ cup extra virgin olive oil
- 1 tbsp. balsamic vinegar
- ⅔ cup fresh lemon juice

Directions

- Combine garlic clove, water, and bouillon cubes in a saucepan; bring the mixture to a gentle boil over medium-low heat.

- Stir in quinoa and simmer, covered, for about 20 minutes or until the water has been absorbed and quinoa is tender.

- Discard garlic clove and transfer the cooked quinoa to a large bowl.

- Stir in olives, onion, chicken, bell pepper, feta cheese, chives, parsley, sea salt, extra virgin olive oil, balsamic vinegar, and lemon juice.

- Serve warm or chilled.

Healthy Greek Salad

Total time: 15 minutes

Prep time: 15 minutes

Cook time: 0 minutes

Yield: 6 servings

Ingredients

- 1 small red onion, chopped

- 2 cucumbers, peeled and chopped

- 3 large ripe tomatoes, chopped

- 4 tsp. freshly squeezed lemon juice

- ¼ cup extra virgin olive oil

- 1 ½ tsp. dried oregano

- Sea salt

- Ground black pepper

- 6 pitted and sliced black Greek olives

- 1 cup crumbled feta cheese

Directions

- Combine onion, cucumber, and tomatoes in a shallow salad bowl; sprinkle with lemon juice, extra virgin olive, oregano, sea salt and black pepper.

- Sprinkle the olives and feta over the salad and serve immediately.

Mediterranean Green Salad

Total time: 25 minutes

Prep time: 15 minutes

Cook time: 10 minutes

Yield: 4 servings

Ingredients

- ½ loaf rustic sourdough bread

- ¼ tsp. paprika

- 2 tbsp. manchego, finely grated

- 7 tbsp. extra virgin olive oil, divided

- 1 ½ tbsp. sherry vinegar

- ½ tsp. sea salt

- 1 tsp. freshly ground black pepper

- 1 tsp. Dijon mustard

- 5 cups mixed baby greens

- ¾ cup green olives, pitted and halved

- 12 thin slices of Serrano ham, roughly chopped

Directions

- Cut the bread into bite-sized cubes and set aside.

- Preheat oven to 400°F.

- In a mixing bowl, combine paprika, manchego and 6 tbsps. of olive oil.

- Add the bread cubes and toss them until they are evenly coated with the flavored oil.

- Arrange the bread on a baking sheet and bake for about 8 minutes until golden brown and let the bread cool.

- In a separate bowl, combine the vinegar, salt, pepper, mustard and the remaining olive oil.

- Add this mixture to a larger bowl containing the greens until they are lightly coated with the vinaigrette.

- Add all the other ingredients and the croutons and toss well.

- Serve the salad on four plates.

- This salad has an amazing taste and leaves you energized to face the remaining part of the day.

Bulgur Salad

Total time: 30 minutes

Prep time: 10 minutes

Cook time: 20 minutes

Yield: 4 servings

Ingredients

- 1 tbsp. unsalted butter

- 2 tbsp. extra virgin olive oil, divided

- 2 cups bulgur

- 4 cups water

- ¼ tsp. sea salt

- 1 medium cucumber, deseeded and chopped

- ¼ cup dill, chopped

- 1 handful black olives, pitted and chopped

- 2 tsp. red wine vinegar

Directions

- Place a saucepan over medium heat and add 1 tbsp. of butter and 1 tbsp. of olive oil.

- Toast the bulgur in the oil until it turns golden brown and starts to crackle.

- Add 4 cups of water to the saucepan and season with the salt.

- Cover the saucepan and simmer until all the water gets absorbed for about 20 minutes.

- In a mixing bowl, combine the chopped cucumber with dill, olives, red wine vinegar and the remaining olive oil.

- Serve this over the bulgur.

Mediterranean Breakfast Recipes

Garlic Scrambled Eggs

Total time: 25 minutes

Prep time: 10 minutes

Cooking time: 15 minutes

Yield: 2 servings

Ingredients

- ½ tsp. extra virgin olive oil

- ½ cup ground beef

- ½ tsp. garlic powder

- 3 eggs

- Salt

- Pepper

Directions

- Set a medium-sized pan over medium heat.

- Add extra virgin olive oil and heat until hot but not smoking.

- Stir in ground beef and cook for about 10 minutes or until almost done.

- Stir in garlic and sauté for about 2 minutes.

- In a large bowl, beat the eggs until almost frothy; season with salt and pepper.

- Add the egg mixture to the pan with the cooked beef and scramble until ready.

- Serve with toasted bread and olives, for a healthy, satisfying breakfast!

Fry Breakfast Stir

Total time: 25 minutes

Prep time: 5 minutes

Cooking time: 20 minutes

Yield: 4 servings

Ingredients

- 1 tbsp. extra virgin olive oil

- 2 green peppers, sliced

- 2 small onions, finely chopped

- 4 tomatoes, chopped

- ½ tsp. sea salt

- 1 egg

Directions

- Heat olive oil in a medium-sized pan over medium-high heat.

- Add green pepper and sauté for about 2 minutes.

- Lower heat to medium and continue cooking, covered, for 3 more minutes.

- Stir in onion and cook for about 2 minutes or until brown.

- Stir in tomatoes and salt; cover and simmer to get a soft juicy mixture.

- In a bowl, beat the egg; drizzle over the tomato mixture and cook for about 1 minute. (Don't stir).

- Serve with chopped cucumbers, feta cheese and black olives for a great breakfast!

Healthy Breakfast Casserole

Total time: 60 minutes

Prep time: 10 minutes

Cooking time: 50 minutes

Yield: 6 servings

Ingredients

- 2 tbsp. extra virgin olive oil, divided

- ½ a medium-sized onion, diced

- 2 medium-sized yellow potatoes. diced

- 1 lb. zucchini, sliced

- 3 portabella mushroom caps, diced

- 150g torn fresh spinach

- 200g ricotta

- 200g light ricotta cheese

- 2 cups of egg whites

- 12 grape tomatoes,sliced into⅓ pieces

- 3 peeled and roasted fresh peppers, sliced

- 2 sourdough rolls

- 4 tbsp. Pecorino Romano cheese, grated

- 100g skim-milk mozzarella cheese, grated

Directions

- Preheat the oven to 400°F.

- Mix together olive oil, onion and potato and roast for at least 15 minutes; remove from oven and keep on the baking tray.

- In a bowl, combine together ½ tablespoon olive oil and zucchini; toss to coat well and transfer to a baking tray.

- Return all the vegetables to oven and roast for about 40 minutes or until golden in color.

- In the meantime, place ½ tablespoon olive oil in a pan and sauté mushrooms for about 4 minutes.

- Remove the cooked mushrooms from pan and set aside.

- Add the remaining olive oil to pan and sauté chopped spinach until tender.

- In a mixing bowl, combine together both types of ricotta and egg whites; set aside. Combine together all the vegetables, including grape tomatoes and peppers, with sourdough rolls in a 9 x 13 baking dish; top with the ricotta mixture and sprinkle with pecorino and mozzarella cheese.

- Bake for at least 40 minutes or until done. Remove from the oven, cool slightly.

- Cut into six slices and enjoy your breakfast.

Yogurt Pancakes Mix

Total time: 15 minutes

Prep time: 10 minutes

Cooking time: 5 minutes

Yield: 5 servings

Ingredients

- Whole-wheat pancake mix

- 1 cup yogurt

- 1 tbsp. baking powder

- 1 tbsp. baking soda

- 1 cup skimmed milk

- 3 whole eggs

- ½ tsp. extra virgin olive oil

Directions

- Combine together whole-wheat pancake mix, yogurt, baking powder, baking soda, skimmed milk and eggs in large bowl.

- Stir until well blended.

- Heat a pan oiled lightly with olive oil.

- Pour ¼ cup batter onto the heated pan and cook for about 2 minutes or until the surface of the pancake has some bubbles.

- Flip and continue cooking until the underside is browned.

- Serve the pancakes warm with a cup of fat-free milk or two tablespoons light maple syrup.

Fruity Nutty Muesli

Total time: 1 hour 15 minutes

Prep time 15 minutes

Cook time 1 hour

Yield: 2 servings

Ingredients

- ⅓ cup almonds, chopped

- ¾ cup oats, toasted

- ½ cup low-fat milk

- ½ cup low-fat Greek yogurt

- ½ green apple, diced

- 2 tbsp. raw honey

Directions

- Preheat oven to 350°F. Place the almonds on a baking sheet and bake until they turn golden brown, about 10 minutes.

- After cooling, mix with the toasted oats, milk and yogurt in a bowl and cover.

- Refrigerate this mixture for an hour until the oats are soft.

- Divide the muesli between two bowls, add the apple and drizzle the honey.

Mediterranean Soup and Stew Recipes

Curried Cauliflower Soup

Total time: 30 minutes

Prep time: 10 minutes

Cook time: 20 minutes

Yields: 4 to 6 servings

Ingredients

- ⅓ cup raw cashews

- ¾ cup water

- 2 tsp. extra virgin olive oil

- 1 medium onion, diced

- 1 can (14-ounce) light coconut milk

- 1 large head cauliflower, chopped in small pieces

- ¼ tsp. ground cinnamon

- 1 tsp. evaporated cane sugar

- 1 tsp. ground turmeric

- 2 tbsp. curry powder

- ¼ cup chopped cilantro

- Caramelized onions

- Salt

Directions

- Blend the cashews in a blender until finely ground.

- Add three-quarters of a cup of water to the cashews and continue blending for 2 more minutes.

- Strain the mixture through a fine mesh strainer into a bowl and set aside.

- Add olive oil to a large pot set over low heat.

- Sauté onions in the hot olive oil until golden brown.

- Add the cashew milk, coconut milk, cauliflower, cinnamon, sugar, turmeric, curry powder and salt.

- Add enough water to cover mixture and bring to a gentle boil.

- Lower the heat and simmer for about 10 minutes or until cauliflower is tender.

- Transfer the mixture to an immersion blender and blend to your desired consistency.

- Return to the pot and heat.

- Ladle the hot soup into bowls and serve garnished with cilantro and onions.

Roasted Veggie Soup

Total time: 1 hour 5 minutes

Prep time: 25 minutes

Cook time: 40 minutes

Yield: 4 servings

Ingredients

- 5 garlic cloves

- 1 tbsp. extra virgin olive oil

- 2 green and yellow bell peppers, diced

- 350 g potatoes, diced

- ½ tsp. chopped rosemary

- 1 large red onion, diced

- 1 yellow zucchini, diced

- 1 ½ cups carrot juice

- 370 g Italian tomatoes, diced

- ½ tsp. chopped rosemary

- 1 tsp. fresh tarragon

Directions

- Preheat your oven to 450°F.

- In a roasting pan, combine garlic and extra virgin olive oil; roast in the preheated oven for about 5 minutes or until oil starts to sizzle.

- Add peppers, potatoes, and rosemary and toss to coat; continue roasting for about 15 minutes more or until potatoes are tender and golden.

- Add onion and yellow zucchini and roast for about 15 minutes more or until zucchini is tender.

- In a saucepan set over medium heat, combine tomatoes, carrot juice, and tarragon; bring to a boil.

- Add the roasted vegetables to the pan; add a small amount of water to the roasting pan and stir, scraping up browned bits that cling to the pan, and add to the saucepan.

- Cook for about 2 minutes or until heated through.

- Serve immediately.

Lemony Soup

Total time: 28 minutes

Prep time: 5 minutes

Cook time: 23 minutes

Yield: 8 servings

Ingredients

- 8 cups low-sodium vegetable or chicken stock

- 2 tbsp. extra virgin olive oil

- ¼ cup flour

- 2 tbsp. butter

- 1 cup orzo

- 4 eggs

- ¾ cup freshly squeezed lemon juice

- Sea salt to taste

- ¼ tsp. ground white pepper

- 8 lemon slices

Directions

- In a soup pot, bring stock to a gentle boil over medium heat; reduce heat to a simmer.

- In a small bowl, mix together extra virgin olive oil, flour and butter.

- Whisk 2 cups of hot stock into the flour mixture until well blended.

- Gradually beat the flour mixture into the pot with stock and simmer for about 10 minutes.

- Stir in orzo and continue cooking for about 5 minutes.

- In the meantime, beat the eggs and lemon juice in a small bowl until well blended and foamy.

- Slowly whisk a cup of hot soup mixture into the egg mixture until well combined.

- Add the egg mixture to the pot with the soup and stir to mix well.

- Simmer for about 10 minutes or until the soup is thick.

- Season with sea salt and pepper and ladle the soup into serving bowl.

- Serve right away garnished with lemon slices.

Cold Cucumber Soup

Total time: 20 minutes + Chilling time

Prep time: 20 minutes

Cook time: 0 minutes

Yields: 4 to 6 servings

Ingredients

- Juice of 1 lemon

- ½ cup chopped fresh parsley

- 2 medium cucumbers

- 1 ½ cups low-sodium chicken broth

- 1 cup fat-free plain yogurt

- 1 1/2 cups fat-free half and half

- Salt and freshly ground black pepper, to taste

- Chopped fresh dill

Directions

- In a blender or food processor, combine together lemon juice, parsley, and cucumbers and puree until smooth.

- Transfer half of the puree to a plate and set aside.

- Combine together yogurt, half and half, and broth in a medium-sized bowl.

- Add half of the yogurt mixture to the pureed mixture in the blender and puree again until well mixed.

- Sprinkle with salt and pepper and refrigerate in a container.

- Repeat the procedure with the remaining yogurt mixture and the puree.

- Stir the soup and garnish with fresh dill to serve.

Red Lentil Bean Soup

Total time: 1 hour

Prep time: 15 minutes

Cook time: 45 minutes

Yield: 4 servings

Ingredients

- 2 cups dried red lentil beans, rinsed

- 2 tbsp. extra virgin olive oil, plus more for drizzling

- 2 large onions, diced

- 1 - 2 finely chopped carrots

- 8 cups chicken stock

- 2 ripe tomatoes, cubed

- 1 tsp. ground cumin

- Sea salt

- Black pepper

- 2 cups fresh spinach

Directions

- Soak lentils for at least 2 hours.

- In a pot set over medium high heat, boil the lentils until almost cooked.

- In a soup pot, heat extra virgin olive oil over medium heat; add diced onions and carrots and sauté for about 4 minutes or until tender.

- Add stock, tomatoes, cumin, sea salt and pepper and simmer for about 40 minutes or until lentils are tender.

- Stir in spinach until just wilted and drizzle with extra virgin olive oil just before serving.

Fish Soup with Rotelle

Total time: 45 minutes

Prep time: 15 minutes

Cook time: 30 minutes

Yield: 4 servings

Ingredients

- 2 tbsp. extra virgin olive oil, plus more for drizzling
- 1 tbsp. minced garlic
- 1 onion, diced
- ½ can crushed tomatoes
- 1 cup rotelle pasta
- ¼ tsp. rosemary
- 1 dozen mussels in their shells
- 1 pound monkfish

Directions

- In a saucepan over medium heat, heat extra virgin olive oil; add garlic and onion and sauté for about 4 minutes or until soft.

- Stir in tomatoes, water, pasta, and rosemary; season with sea salt and pepper and cook for about 15 minutes.

- Clean mussels and cut monkfish into small pieces; stir into the soup and simmer for about 10 minutes more, or until all mussel shells open.

- Discard unopened shells and serve soup drizzled with more extra virgin olive oil, with crusty bread.

Mediterranean Seafood Recipes

Grilled Salmon

Total time: 23 minutes

Prep time: 15 minutes

Cook time: 8 minutes

Yield: 4 servings

Ingredients

- 2 tbsp. freshly squeezed lemon juice
- 1 tbsp. minced garlic
- 1 tbsp. chopped fresh parsley
- 4 tbsp. chopped fresh basil
- 4 salmon fillets, each 5 ounces
- Extra virgin olive oil?
- Sea salt and cracked black pepper, to taste
- 4 green olives, chopped
- Cracked black pepper
- 4 thin slices lemon

Directions

- Lightly coat grill rack with olive oil cooking spray and position it 4 inches from heat; heat grill to medium high.

- Combine lemon juice, minced garlic, parsley and basil in a small bowl.

- Coat fish with extra virgin olive oil and season with sea salt and pepper.

- Top each fish fillet with equal amount of garlic mixture and place on the heated grill, herb-side down.

- Grill over high heat for about 4 minutes or until the edges turn white; turn over and transfer the fish to aluminum foil.

- Reduce heat and continue grilling for about 4 minutes more.

- Transfer the grilled fish to plates and garnish with lemon slices and green olives.

- Serve immediately.

Grilled Tuna

Total time: 1 hour 16 minutes

Prep time: 10 minutes

Chill time: 1 hour

Cook time: 6 minutes

Yield: 4 servings

Ingredients

- 4 tuna steaks, 1 inch thick

- 3 tbsp. extra virgin oil

- ½ cup hickory wood chips, soaked

- Sea salt

- Freshly ground black pepper

- Juice of 1 lime

Directions

- Place tuna and the olive oil in a zip lock plastic bag, seal and refrigerate for an hour.

- Prepare a charcoal or gas grill.

- When using a coal grill, scatter a handful of hickory wood chips when the coals are hot for added flavor.

- Lightly grease the grill grate.

- Season the tuna with salt and pepper and cook on the grill for about 6 minutes, turning only once.

- Transfer to a plate.

- Drizzle the lime juice over the fish and serve immediately.

Spanish Cod

Total time: 35 minutes

Prep time: 20 minutes

Cook time: 15 minutes

Yield: 6 servings

Ingredients

- 1 tbsp. extra virgin olive oil

- 1 tbsp. butter

- ¼ cup onion, finely chopped

- 2 tbsp. garlic, chopped

- 1 cup tomato sauce

- 15 cherry tomatoes, halved

- ¼ cup deli marinated Italian vegetable salad, drained and chopped

- ½ cup green olives, chopped

- 1 dash cayenne pepper

- 1 dash black pepper

- 1 dash paprika

- 6 cod fillets

Directions

- Place a large skillet over medium heat and add the olive oil and butter.

- Add the onion and garlic and cook until garlic starts browning.

- Add the tomato sauce and tomatoes and let them simmer.

- Stir in the marinated vegetables, olives and spices.

- Cook the fillet in the sauce for 8 minutes over medium heat.

- Serve immediately.

Mediterranean Cod

Total time: 50 minutes

Prep time: 15 minutes

Cook time: 35 minutes

Yield: 4 servings

Ingredients

- 1 tbsp. extra virgin olive oil

- 100g frozen chopped onion

- 1 tbsp. frozen chopped garlic

- 230g can Italian tomatoes, chopped

- 1 tbsp. tomato purée

- 400g pack skinless and boneless cod fillets

- 200g frozen mixed peppers

- 1 tbsp. chopped frozen parsley

- 50g pitted black olives

- 800g package frozen white rice

Directions

- Add extra virgin olive oil to a saucepan set over medium heat; stir in onion and sauté for about 3 minutes.

- Add garlic and sauté for 2 minutes more or until fragrant.

- Stir in the tomatoes, tomato puree, and water and bring to a gentle boil.

- Reduce heat and simmer for about 20 minutes or until thickened.

- Add cod and peppers; nudge the fish in the sauce a bit and bring back to a boil; lower heat and simmer for about 8 minutes.

- Sprinkle with parsley and olives and simmer for 2 minutes more.

- In the meantime, follow package instructions to cook rice.

- Serve fish with hot rice.

Easy Fish Dish

Total time: 45 minutes

Prep time: 15 minutes

Cook time: 30 minutes

Yields: 4 servings

Ingredients

- 4 fillets halibut (6 ounces)

- 1 tbsp. Greek seasoning

- 1 tbsp. lemon juice

- ¼ cup olive oil

- ¼ cup capers

- 1 jar (5 ounce) pitted Kalamata olives

- 1 chopped onion

- 1 large tomato, chopped

- A pinch of freshly ground black pepper

- A pinch of salt

Directions

- Preheat your oven to 250°F.

- Arrange the halibut fillets onto an aluminum foil sheet and sprinkle with Greek seasoning.

- In a bowl, combine together lemon juice, olive oil, capers, olives, onion, tomato, salt and pepper; spoon the mixture over the fillets and fold the edges of the foil to seal.

- Place the folded foil onto a baking sheet and bake for about 40 minutes or until the fish flakes easily when touched with a fork.

Baked Fish

Total time: 1 hour

Prep time: 10 minutes

Cook time: 50 minutes

Yields: 4 servings

Ingredients

- 2 tsp. extra virgin olive oil
- 1 large sliced onion
- 1 tbsp. orange zest
- ¼ cup orange juice
- ¼ cup lemon juice
- ¾ cup apple juice
- 1 minced clove garlic
- 1 (16 oz.) can whole tomatoes, drained and coarsely chopped, the juice reserved
- ½ cup reserved tomato juice
- 1 bay leaf
- ½ tsp. crushed dried basil
- ½ tsp. crushed dried thyme
- ½ tsp. crushed dried oregano
- 1 tsp. crushed fennel seeds
- A pinch of black pepper
- 1 lb. fish fillets (perch, flounder or sole)

Directions

- Add oil to a large nonstick skillet set over medium heat.

- Sauté the onion in the oil for about 5 minutes or until tender.

- Stir in all the remaining ingredients except the fish.

- Simmer uncovered for about 30 minutes.

- Arrange the fish in a baking dish and cover with the sauce.

- Bake the fish at 375°F, uncovered, for about 15 minutes or until it flakes easily when tested with a fork.

Mediterranean Meat Recipes

Parmesan Meat Loaf

Total time: 1 hour

Prep time: 10 minutes

Cook time: 50 minutes

Yield: 4 servings

Ingredients

- 1½ pounds ground beef

- ½ cup bread crumbs

- ½ cup chopped flat-leaf parsley

- 1 grated onion

- 1 large egg

- ½ cup grated Parmesan

- ¼ cup tomato paste

- Sea salt

- Freshly ground black pepper

Directions

- Preheat your oven to 400°F. In a large bowl, mix together ground beef, bread crumbs, parsley, onion, egg, Parmesan cheese, tomato paste, sea salt and pepper.

- Line a baking sheet with foil and add the beef mixture, pressing to form an 8-inch loaf.

- Bake in the preheated oven for about 50 minutes or until cooked through.

Mediterranean Beef Pitas

Total time: 15 minutes

Prep time: 10 minutes

Cook time: 5 minutes

Yield: 4 servings

Ingredients

- 1pound ground beef

- Freshly ground black pepper

- Sea salt

- 1 ½ tsp. dried oregano

- 2 tbsp. extra virgin olive oil, divided

- ¼ small red onion, sliced

- 3/4cup store-bought hummus

- 2 tbsp. fresh flat-leaf parsley

- 4 pitas

- 4 lemon wedges

Directions

- Form beef into 16 patties; season with ¼ teaspoon ground pepper, ½ teaspoon sea salt and oregano.

- Add 1 tablespoon of extra virgin olive oil in a skillet set over medium heat; cook the beef patties for about 2 minutes per side or until lightly browned.

- To serve, top pitas with the beef patties, hummus, parsley and onion and drizzle with the remaining extra virgin olive oil; garnish with lemon wedges.

Seasoned Lamb Burgers

Total time: 30 minutes

Prep time: 20 minutes

Cook time: 10 minutes

Yield: 4 servings

Ingredients

- 1 ½ pounds ground lamb
- 1 tsp. ground cumin
- ½ tsp. ground cinnamon
- 1 tsp. ground ginger
- ¼ cup extra virgin olive oil, divided
- 1 tsp. black pepper, freshly ground; divided
- ¼ cup fresh cilantro
- 2 tbsp. fresh oregano
- 1 small clove garlic, pressed
- ¾ tsp. red pepper flakes, crushed
- ¼ cup fresh flat leaf parsley
- 1 tbsp. sherry vinegar
- 2 pitas, warmed and halved
- Sliced tomato
- 1 8 oz of package plain Greek yogurt

Directions

- Prepare a charcoal or gas grill fire.

- Mix the ground lamb with cumin, cinnamon, ginger, 1 tablespoon extra virgin olive oil and ½ teaspoon black pepper.

- Mix well and divide this into four burgers.

- Spray the grill with some olive oil and grill the burgers for 5 minutes on each side.

- Combine the rest of the olive oil, cilantro, oregano, garlic, red pepper flakes, parsley and vinegar in a food processor until it forms a thick paste.

- Serve each burger in pita bread on a plate with sliced tomato, the processed sauce and a serving of yogurt.

Mediterranean Flank Steak

Total time: 1 hour

Prep time: 20 minutes

Cook time: 40 minutes

Yield: 4 to 6 servings

Ingredients

- 2 tbsp. chopped aromatic herbs (marjoram, rosemary, sage, thyme, or a mix)

- 2 cloves garlic, minced

- 2 tbsp. extra virgin olive oil

- 1 tbsp. sea salt

- 1 tbsp. ground black pepper

- 1½- to 2-lb. flank steak, trimmed

- ½ cup Greek vinaigrette

Directions

- In a small bowl, mix together herbs, garlic, extra virgin olive oil, sea salt, and pepper; rub over the steak and let rest for about 20 minutes.

- In the meantime, heat your gas grill to medium high.

- Grill the steak for about 15 minutes, turning meat every 4 minutes for even cooking.

- Transfer the cooked steak to a cutting board and let rest for about 5 minutes; slice into small slices and place on plates.

- Drizzle with vinaigrette and serve immediately.

Healthy Beef and Broccoli

Total time: 25 minutes

Prep time: 5 minutes

Cook time: 20 minutes

Ingredients

- 8ml vegetable oil, divided
- 100g flank steak, thinly sliced
- 7.5g corn starch
- 90g broccoli florets
- 60ml water
- 1 green onion, thinly sliced
- 1/2 shallots, finely chopped
- 1 small cloves garlic, minced
- 1g crushed red pepper flakes
- 1g minced fresh ginger
- 5ml honey
- 20 ml soy sauce

Directions

- Add oil to a skillet set over medium heat.

- Stir in beef and cook for about 8 minutes or until browned.

- Remove the beef from the pan and set aside.

- Add green onions, shallots and garlic to the same pan and cook for 1 minute, stirring.

- Stir in broccoli and cook for about 5 minutes.

- Combine cornstarch and water in a mixing bowl until well blended.

- In a separate bowl, combine red pepper flakes, ginger, honey, and soy sauce; stir in the cornstarch mixture until well combined.

- Add sauce to the pan and cook for about 5 minutes or until thick.

- Stir in beef and cook for about 3 minutes.

- Serve over brown rice.

Grilled Sage Lamb Kabob

Total time: 4 hours, 50 minutes

Marinating time: 4 hours

Prep time: 20 minutes

Cook time: 30 minutes

Yield: 2 servings

Ingredients

- 1 tbsp. fresh lemon juice
- 2 tbsp. fresh chives
- 2 tbsp. fresh flat leaf parsley
- 2 tbsp. fresh sage
- 1 tbsp. dark brown sugar
- 1 tbsp. extra virgin olive oil
- 2 tbsp. dry sherry
- 1 tbsp. pure maple syrup
- ¼ tsp. sea salt
- 8 ounces lean lamb shoulder
- 2 cups water
- 4 medium red potatoes
- White onion, cut into halves
- 6 shitake mushroom caps
- ½ red bell pepper

Directions

- In a blender, combine together lemon juice, chives, parsley, sage, brown sugar, extra virgin olive oil, sherry, maple syrup, and salt; puree until very smooth.

- Cut lamb into 8 cubes and add to a zipper bag along with the marinade; marinate in the refrigerator for at least 4 hours.

- Bring a pot with water to a rolling boil.

- Cut potatoes in halves and add to the pot along with half onion; steam for about 15 minutes. Remove from heat and let cool.

- Chop the remaining onion and pepper.

- On a skewer, alternate lamb cube, mushroom cap, pepper, onion and potato.

- Reserve the marinade.

- Grill the kabobs over hot grill, turning every 3 minutes and basting with the reserved marinade.

Vegetarian Mediterranean Recipes

Vegan Bruschetta

Total time: 10 minutes

Prep time: 5 minutes

Cook time: 5 minutes

Yields: 12 servings

Ingredients

- 1 tsp. balsamic vinegar

- ½ tsp. minced garlic

- 2 tomatoes, sliced

- A pinch of ground black pepper

- 8 fresh basil leaves

- 12 (½ inch) slices Italian bread

Directions

- Combine together all the topping ingredients and spread evenly over each bread slice.

- Toast at 375 °F for a few minutes or until crisp.

- Enjoy!

Stuffed Grape Leaves Dish

Total time: 2 hours

Prep time: 30 minutes

Cook time: 1 hour 30 minutes

Yield: 8 servings

Ingredients

- 30 fresh grape leaves

- 2 tbsp. extra virgin olive oil

- 2 cups finely diced onion

- 1 cup brown rice

- 1 cup dried currants or raisins

- 1 cup chopped fresh mint

- 1 cup chopped fresh parsley

- 1 cup chopped hulled pistachios

- 2 cups tomato juice

- Sea salt and pepper, to taste

- Pomegranate molasses, to drizzle

- ¼ cup freshly squeezed lemon juice

- 1 lemon, sliced

- 1 tsp. extra virgin olive oil for brushing casserole dish and top of casserole

Directions

- Place grape leaves in a pot of boiling water; cook for about 2 minutes and remove from heat; drain, and set aside.
- In a large saucepan set over medium heat, heat extra virgin olive oil; add onion, and sauté for about 10 minutes or until lightly browned.
- Stir in rice and 2 ½ cups of water; bring to a gentle boil, cover and reduce heat to medium low.
- Cook for about 40 minutes or until rice is cooked through and water is absorbed.
- Remove the cooked rice from heat and stir in lemon juice, raisins, mint, parsley, pistachios, tomato juice, sea salt, and pepper.
- Preheat your oven to 350°F.
- Grease a 2-quart baking dish with extra virgin olive oil and line its bottom with grape leaves, allowing them to hang over the sides.
- With paper towels, pat the leaves dry and spread with half of the rice mixture.
- Top the rice mixture with more grape leaves and top with the remaining rice.
- Cover with the remaining leaves and fold over the leaves around edges to seal.
- Brush the top with extra virgin olive oil and bake in the preheated oven for about 40 minutes or until casserole is firm and dry and the grape leaves darken.
- Using a wet knife, cut the casserole into eight pieces and place each on eight plates.
- Drizzle each serving with pomegranate molasses and garnish with lemon slices.

Tomato and Spinach Pasta

Total time: 35 minutes

Prep time: 10 minutes

Cook time: 25 minutes

Ingredients

- 100g whole-wheat pasta

- 7.5ml extra virgin olive oil

- ½ onion, sliced

- 60g can tomatoes, drained

- 60g frozen spinach

- ⅓ cup crumbled feta cheese

- 1g salt

- 1g ground pepper

Directions

- Follow package instructions to cook pasta in a pot of boiling water until al dente.

- In the meantime, add oil to a skillet set over medium heat; stir in onion and sauté for 3 minutes. Stir in tomatoes and simmer for about 10 minutes.

- Add spinach and cook until heated through.

- Drain the cooked pasta and toss with the sauce until well coated.

- Season with salt and pepper and serve topped with feta.

Grilled Veggies Tagine

Total time: 1 hour

Prep time: 10 minutes

Cook time: 50 minutes

Yield: 6 servings

Ingredients

- ¼ cup golden raisins
- 6 small red potatoes, cut in quarters
- ¼ cup pine nuts, toasted
- 2/3 cup couscous, uncooked
- 2 garlic cloves, pressed
- I medium red onion, wedged
- 1 tsp. fennel seeds, crushed
- ¼ tsp. cinnamon, ground
- 1 ¾ cups onions, chopped
- 1 tsp. extra virgin olive oil
- 1 tsp. cumin, ground
- ¼ cup green olives, pitted and chopped
- 1 ½ cups water
- ¼ tsp. freshly ground black pepper
- Cooking spray
- 2 red bell peppers, diced
- 1 green bell pepper, diced
- ½ tsp. kosher salt
- 2 tsp. balsamic vinegar
- ½ can tomatoes, chopped

Directions

- Prepare a gas or charcoal grill.

- Combine the bell peppers, red onion, and ¼ teaspoon sea salt, vinegar and ½ teaspoon olive oil in a zip lock plastic bag and toss well.

- Place a large non-stick saucepan on medium heat and add the remaining olive oil and add the garlic and chopped onion.

- Sauté these for about 3 minutes and add fennel, cumin and cinnamon.

- Let them cook for a further 1 minute then add the remaining salt, olives, raisins, potatoes, tomatoes, black pepper and water and bring the pan to a boil.

- Cover the saucepan, and simmer for 25 minutes or until the potatoes are tender

- Remove the onions and bell peppers from the plastic bag and grill on a rack coated with cooking spray for about 10 minutes.

- Boil the remaining water in a separate saucepan and slowly stir in the couscous.

- Remove from heat and cover the pan and let it stand for 5 minutes.

- Serve the tomato mixture over couscous and top with the grilled onions, bell peppers and pine nuts.

Olive, Bell Pepper and Arugula Salsa

Total time: 30 minutes

Prep time: 25 minutes

Cook time: 5 minutes

Yield: 1 ½ cups

Ingredients

- 1 ½ tbsp. extra virgin olive oil

- 1 tsp. crushed fennel seeds

- 1 red and 1 yellow bell peppers, diced

- 16 pitted Kalamata olives, chopped

- Sea salt and pepper, to taste

- ½ cup chopped baby arugula

Directions

- In a large nonstick skillet, heat extra virgin olive oil; sauté fennel seeds for about 1 minute, stirring.

- Stir in bell peppers and continue sautéing for 4 minutes more or until peppers are tender.

- Scrape the pepper mixture into a bowl; stir in olives, sea salt, and pepper.

- Let stand for at least 2 minutes, stirring occasionally, for flavors to meld.

- Add in arugula, toss until slightly wilted, and serve.

Mediterranean Pizza Recipes

Turkish-Style Pizza

Total time: 45 minutes

Prep time: 30 minutes

Cook time: 15 minutes

Yield: 1 14 by 9-inch pizza

Ingredients

- 1 tsp. extra virgin-olive oil, plus 1 tbsp., divided

- Cornmeal, for dusting

- 12 ounces whole-wheat pizza dough

- 1 ½ cups grated Monterey Jack cheese or fontina

- 1 cup diced sweet onion

- 1 ½ cups diced tomatoes

- 2 tbsp. minced seeded jalapeno pepper

- 2 ounces sliced pastrami, diced

- Freshly ground pepper

- ⅓ cup fresh flat-leaf parsley, chopped

Directions

- Position an inverted baking sheet on the lower oven rack and preheat to 500°F.

- Lightly oil a large baking sheet and dust with the cornmeal.

- Lightly flour a clean work surface and roll the dough into 10×15-inch oval.

- Transfer the rolled dough to the baking sheet and fold edges under to form a rim.

- Brush the rim with about 1 teaspoon of extra virgin olive oil.

- Sprinkle the crust with grated cheese, leaving about ½-inch border and top with onion, tomatoes, jalapeno, pastrami, and pepper.

- Drizzle with the remaining extra virgin oil and bake in the preheated oven for about 14 minutes or until the bottom is golden and crisp.

- Serve the pizza warm sprinkled with chopped parsley.

Mediterranean Veggie Pizza

Total time: 27 minutes

Prep time: 15 minutes

Cook time: 12 minutes

Yield: 4 servings

Ingredients

- 1 tbsp. cornmeal

- 1 can refrigerated pizza dough

- 2 tbsp. commercial pesto

- ½ cup mozzarella cheese, shredded

- 1 pack frozen artichoke hearts, thawed, drained and coarsely chopped

- 1 ounce prosciutto, thinly sliced

- 2 tbsp. Parmesan, shredded

- 1 ½ cups Arugula leaves

- 1 ½ tbsp. fresh lemon juice

- Cooking spray

Directions

- Preheat your oven to 500°F.

- Meanwhile, coat a baking sheet with cooking spray and sprinkle with cornmeal.

- Place the dough on the baking sheet by rolling it out.

- Evenly spread the pesto on the dough leaving out close to half an inch from the edge.

- Add the mozzarella over the pesto and now put the baking sheet on the bottom rack of the oven and bake for 5 minutes.

- Add the artichokes onto the pizza plus prosciutto and Parmesan then return the baking sheet to the oven and bake for another 5 – 6 minutes.

- In a small bowl, mix the arugula and the lemon juice and use this to top the pizza.

- You are ready to serve.

Mediterranean Smoothies

Berry Bliss

Total time: 5 minutes

Yields: 2 servings

Ingredients:

- 2 cups plain low-fat Greek yogurt

- 1 tbsp. flaxseed

- 2 tbsp. almond butter

- 1 cup frozen blueberries

- 1 cup frozen strawberries

- 1 frozen banana

Directions:

- Combine all ingredients in a blender and blend until smooth.

Pumpkin Smoothie

Total time: 15 minutes

Yield: 2 servings

Ingredients

- ½ cup skim milk

- ½ cup ice, crushed

- ½ cup pumpkin butter

- ⅓ cup of low-fat Greek yogurt

- 2 tsps. maple syrup

- ½ tsp. cinnamon

- 2 tsp. vanilla extract

Directions

- Combine all ingredients in a blender and blend until smooth.

- Serve in a tall glass with a straw.

Skinny Smoothie

Total time: 5 minutes

Yields: 2 servings

Ingredients

- ½ cup freshly squeezed tangerine or orange juice

- ½ cup honeydew chunks

- ½ banana, chopped

- 1 kiwi, peeled and thinly chopped

- ½ cup frozen non-fat plain Greek yogurt or frozen kefir

- 1 cup baby spinach

- ¼ cup fresh mint leaves, plus extra sprigs for garnish

Directions

- Combine everything in a blender and blend until smooth and creamy.

- Serve in two tall glasses and garnish with a mint sprig.

Mango Smoothie Surprise

Total time: 5 minutes

Yields: 1 serving

Ingredients

- 1 tbsp. lime juice (freshly squeezed)

- ¼ cup nonfat vanilla yogurt

- ½ cup fresh mango juice

- ¼ cup mashed avocado

- ¼ cup diced mango

- ½ tbsp. honey

- 6 ice cubes

Directions

- Combine all the ingredients in a blender and blend on high until smooth.

- Pour in a tall serving glass and garnish with a strawberry or mango slice, if desired. Enjoy!

Oat-Berry Smoothie

Total time: 5 minutes

Yields: 2 servings

Ingredients

- ½ cup oats

- 1 cup nonfat plan Greek yogurt

- 1 cup unsweetened almond milk

- ½ banana

- ½ cup berries

Directions

- Combine all ingredients in a blender and blend until very smooth. Enjoy!

Banana Blueberry Blast

Total time: 5 minutes

Yields: 2 servings

Ingredients

- 1 ½ cups plain nonfat Greek yogurt

- 1 cup blueberries

- 1 banana

- 5 walnuts

- ½ cup oats

Directions

- Add all the ingredients to a blender and blend until very smooth. Enjoy!

Mediterranean Appetizers

Mango Salsa

Total time: 20 minutes

Prep time: 20 minutes

Cook time: 0 minutes

Yield: 4 servings

Ingredients

- 1 cup cucumber, chopped

- 2 cups mango, diced

- ½ cup cilantro, minced

- 2 tbsp. fresh lime juice

- 1 tbsp. scallions, minced

- ¼ tsp. chipotle powder

- ¼ tsp. sea salt

Directions

- Mix together all ingredients in a bowl and serve or refrigerate.

Roasted Beet Muhammara

Total time: 1 hour 20 minutes

Prep time: 20 minutes

Cook time: 1 hour

Yield: 1 ½ Cups

Ingredients

- 9 oz. trimmed and rinsed red beets

- ¼ cup plus 1 tbsp. extra virgin olive oil, divided

- 1 ½ tsp. freshly squeezed lemon juice

- 1 ½ tbsp. pomegranate molasses

- ½ cup sliced scallions

- 3/4 cup lightly toasted walnuts

- 1 tsp. ground cumin

- 1 tsp. Aleppo pepper

- Sea salt

Directions

- Place a rack in the center of oven and preheat to 375°F.

- Place beets in a baking dish and rub with 1 tablespoon extra virgin olive oil and cover with foil.

- Roast in the preheated oven for about 1 hour or until tender.

- Remove from oven and let cool; peel and then chop to yield 1 cup.

- In a food processor, pulse together the beets, scallions, and walnuts until finely chopped.

- Add lemon juice, pomegranate molasses, cumin, pepper, ½ teaspoon sea salt and the remaining extra virgin olive oil; process until very smooth.

- Adjust seasoning to your liking and serve cold or at room temperature.

Roasted Asparagus

Total time: 15 minutes

Prep time: 5 minutes

Cook time: 10 minutes

Yield: 4 servings

Ingredients

- 1 pound fresh asparagus

- 1 tbsp. extra virgin olive oil

- 1 medium lemon

- 1/2 tsp. freshly grated nutmeg

- 1/2 tsp. kosher salt

- ½ tsp. black pepper

Directions

- Preheat your oven to 500°F.

- Arrange asparagus on an aluminum foil and drizzle with extra virgin olive oil; toss until well coated.

- Spread the asparagus in a single layer and fold the edges of foil to make a tray.

- Roast the asparagus in the oven for about 5 minutes; toss and continue roasting for 5 minutes more or until browned.

- Sprinkle the roasted asparagus with nutmeg, salt, zest and pepper to serve.

Fig Tapenade

Total time: 15 minutes

Prep time: 15 minutes

Cook time: 0 minutes

Yields: 16 servings

Ingredients

- 1 cup dried figs

- ½ cup water

- 1 cup Kalamata olives

- 1 tbsp. chopped fresh thyme

- ½ tsp. balsamic vinegar

- 1 tbsp. extra virgin olive oil

Directions

- Pulse the figs in a food processor until well chopped; add water and continue pulsing to form a paste. Add olives and pulse until well blended.

- Add thyme, vinegar, and extra virgin olive oil and pulse until very smooth.

- Serve with walnut crackers.

Squash Fries

Total time: 25 minutes

Prep time: 15 minutes

Cook time: 10 minutes

Yields: 6 servings

Ingredients

- 1 medium butternut squash

- 1 tbsp. extra virgin olive oil

- ½ tbsp. Grapeseed oil?

- ⅛ tsp. sea salt

Directions

- Peel and remove seeds from the squash; cut into thin slices and place them in a bowl.

- Coat with extra virgin olive oil and grapeseed oil; sprinkle with salt and toss to coat well.

- Arrange the squash slices onto three baking sheets and broil in the oven until crispy.

Healthy Spiced Nuts

Total time: 20 minutes

Prep time: 10 minutes

Cook time: 10 minutes

Yields: 4 servings

Ingredients

- ⅔ cup walnuts

- ⅔ cup pecans

- ⅔ cup almonds

- ½ tsp. black pepper

- ½ tsp. cumin

- 1 tsp. chili powder

- ½ tsp. sea salt

- 1 tbsp. extra virgin olive oil

Directions

- Put the nuts in a skillet set over medium heat and toast until lightly browned.

- In the meantime, prepare the spice mixture; combine black pepper, cumin, chili powder, and salt in a bowl.

- Coat the toasted nuts with extra virgin olive oil and sprinkle with the spice mixture to serve.

Mediterranean Poultry Recipes

Chicken and Penne

Total time: 50 minutes

Prep time: 20 minutes

Cook time: 30 minutes

Yield: 4 servings

Ingredients

- 1 package penne pasta

- 1 ½ tbsp. butter

- ½ cup red onion, chopped

- 2 cloves garlic, pressed

- ¾ kg chicken breasts, deboned and skinned, cut in halves

- 1 can artichoke hearts, soaked in water, chopped

- ½ cup feta cheese, crumbled

- 2 tbsp. lemon juice

- 1 tomato, chopped

- 3 tbsp. fresh parsley, chopped

- Sea salt

- Freshly ground black pepper

- 1 tsp. oregano, dried

Directions

- Cook the penne pasta until al dente in a large saucepan with salted boiling water.

- Melt butter in a large skillet over medium heat and add the onions and garlic.

- Cook these for 2 minutes and add the chicken.

- Stir occasionally until the chicken is golden brown for about 6 minutes.

- Drain the artichoke hearts and add them to the skillet together with the cheese, lemon juice, tomatoes, oregano, parsley and drained pasta.

- Reduce the heat to medium low and cook for 3 minutes.

- Add the salt and pepper to taste and serve warm.

Chicken Salad with Pine Nuts, Raisins and Fennel

Total time: 10 minutes

Prep time: 10 minutes

Cook time: 0 minutes

Chill time: 1 hour

Yield: 1 large bowl

Ingredients
For the dressing:

- 1 tbsp. extra virgin olive oil

- 3 tbsp. mayonnaise

- ½ small clove garlic, mashed with sea salt

- Pinch cayenne

- 1 tbsp. freshly squeezed fresh lemon juice

For the salad:

- 3 tbsp. chopped sweet onion

- ⅓ cup small-diced fresh fennel

- 1 cup shredded cooked chicken

- 2 tbsp. golden raisins

- 2 tbsp. toasted pine nuts

- 2 tbsp. chopped fresh flat-leaf parsley

- Sea salt

- Freshly ground pepper

Directions

- Combine extra virgin olive oil, mayonnaise, garlic, cayenne, and lemon juice in a small bowl; mix well.

- In a separate bowl, mix onion, fennel, chicken, raisins, pine nuts, and parsley; gently add in the dressing and fold the ingredients together.

- Season with sea salt and pepper and refrigerate for at least 1 hour for flavors to meld before serving.

Chicken Stew

Total time: 35 minutes

Prep time: 20 minutes

Cook time: 15 minutes

Yield: 4 servings

Ingredients

- 1 tbsp. extra virgin olive oil

- 3 chicken breast halves (8 ounces each), boneless, skinless, cut into small pieces

- Sea salt

- Freshly ground pepper

- 1 medium onion, sliced

- 4 garlic cloves, sliced

- ½ tsp. dried oregano

- 1 ½ pounds escarole, ends trimmed, chopped

- 1 cup whole-wheat couscous, cooked

- 1 (28 ounces) can whole peeled tomatoes, pureed

Directions

- In a large heavy pot or Dutch oven, heat extra virgin olive oil over medium high heat.

- Rub chicken with sea salt and pepper.

- In batches, cook chicken in olive oil, tossing occasionally, for about 5 minutes or until browned; transfer to a plate and set aside.

- Add onion, garlic and oregano, tomatoes, sea salt and pepper to the pot and cook for about 10 minutes or until onion is lightly browned.

- Add the chicken and cook, covered for about 4 minutes or until opaque.

- Fill the pot with escarole and cook for about 4 minutes or until tender.

- Serve the chicken stew over couscous.

Grilled Turkey with Salsa

Total time: 50 minutes
Prep time: 15 minutes
Cook time: 35 minutes
Yield: 6 servings

Ingredients
For the spice rub:

- 1 ½ tsp. garlic powder
- 1 ½ tsp. sweet paprika
- 2 tsp. crushed fennel seeds
- 2 tsp. dark brown sugar
- 1 tsp. sea salt
- 1 ½ tsp. freshly ground black pepper

For the salsa:

- 2 tbsp. drained capers
- ¼ cup pimento-stuffed green olives, chopped
- 2 scant cups cherry tomatoes, diced
- 1 ½ tbsp. extra virgin olive oil
- 1 large clove garlic, minced
- 2 tbsp. torn fresh basil leaves
- 2 tsp. fresh lemon juice
- ½ tsp. finely grated lemon zest
- 6 turkey breast cutlets
- 1 cup diced red onion
- Sea salt
- Freshly ground black pepper

Directions

- Mix together garlic powder, paprika, fennel seeds, brown sugar, salt and pepper in a small bowl.

- In another bowl, combine capers, olives, tomatoes, onion extra virgin olive oil, garlic, basil, lemon juice and zest, ¼ teaspoon sea salt and pepper; set aside.

- Grill the meat on medium high heat after dipping in the spice rub for about 3 minutes per side or until browned on both sides.

- Transfer the grilled turkey to a serving plate and let rest for about 5 minutes.

- Serve with salsa.

Warm Chicken Avocado Salad

Total time: 35 minutes

Prep time: 15 minutes

Cook time: 20 minutes

Yield: 4 servings

Ingredients

- 2 tbsp. extra virgin olive oil, divided

- 500g chicken breast fillets

- 1 large avocado, peeled, diced

- 2 garlic cloves, sliced

- 1 tsp. ground turmeric

- 3 tsp. ground cumin

- 1 small head broccoli, chopped

- 1 large carrot, diced

- 1/3 cup currants

- 1 1/2 cups chicken stock

- 1 1/2 cups couscous

- Pinch of sea salt

Directions

- In a large frying pan set over medium heat, heat 1 tablespoon extra virgin olive oil; add chicken and cook for about 6 minutes per side or until cooked through; transfer to a plate and keep warm.

- In the meantime, combine currants and couscous in a heatproof bowl; stir in boiling stock and set aside, covered, for at least 5 minutes or until liquid is absorbed.

- With a fork, separate the grains.

- Add the remaining oil to a frying pan and add carrots; cook, stirring, for about 1 minute.

- Stir in broccoli for about 1 minute; stir in garlic, turmeric, and cumin.

- Cook for about 1 minute more and remove the pan from heat.

- Slice the chicken into small slices and add to the broccoli mixture; toss to combine; season with sea salt and serve with the avocado sprinkled on top.

Delicious Mediterranean Chicken

Total time: 55 minutes

Prep time: 25 minutes

Cook time: 30 minutes

Yield: 6 servings

Ingredients

- 2 tsp. extra virgin olive oil

- ½ cup white wine, divided

- 6 chicken breasts, skinned and deboned

- 3 cloves garlic, pressed

- ½ cup onion, chopped

- 3 cups tomatoes, chopped

- ½ cup Kalamata olives

- ¼ cup fresh parsley, chopped

- 2 tsp. fresh thyme, chopped

- Sea salt to taste

Directions

- Heat the oil and 3 tablespoons of white wine in a skillet over medium heat.

- Add the chicken and cook for about 6 minutes on each side until golden.

- Remove the chicken and put it on a plate.

- Add garlic and onions in the skillet and sauté for about 3 minutes and add the tomatoes.

- Let them cook for five minutes then lower the heat and add the remaining white wine and simmer for 10 minutes.

- Add the thyme and simmer for a further 5 minutes.

- Return the chicken to the skillet and cook on low heat until the chicken is well done.

- Add olives and parsley and cook for 1 more minute.

- Add the salt and pepper and serve.

Mediterranean Desserts

Fig Ice Cream

Total time: 1 hour

Prep time: 15 minutes

Cook time: 45 minutes

Yield: 4 servings

Ingredients

- ½ cup ripe figs, stems removed

- ⅓ cup sugar, plus 2 tbsp. sugar

- ⅓ cup honey

- 2 cups half-and-half

- 1 tsp. anise seed

- 3 eggs, separated

- 1 cup crème fraiche

Directions

- Place the figs in a food processor and process until it forms a puree and transfer this to a skillet containing ⅓ cup sugar.

- Cook over medium heat, stirring constantly so that it doesn't stick, for about 30 minutes until it forms a sort of jam.

- In a separate saucepan, heat the honey, half-and-half, and anise seed and bring to a boil. Stir constantly until the honey dissolves.

- Whisk a bit of the hot cream into the egg yolks, pour them into the pan, and continue stirring until the mixture thickens and coats the spoon.

- Transfer this to a bowl and pour in the fig mixture and crème fraiche and chill.

- Whisk the egg whites together with the remaining 2 tbsp. sugar until soft peaks form.

- Fold this into the fig mixture and put in an ice cream maker, following the instructions of the ice cream maker.

- Serve when ready.

Grape Delight

Total time: 20 minutes

Prep time: 20 minutes

Cook time: 0 minutes

Refrigerator time: 1 hour

Yield: 8 servings

Ingredients

- ¾ kg red seedless grapes, washed and drained

- ¾ kg green seedless grapes, washed and drained

- ¼ cup light cream cheese, softened

- ⅓ cup low-fat Greek yogurt

- 1 tsp. vanilla extract

- 2 tbsp. brown sugar

- ½ cup pecans, chopped

- ¼ cup sugar

Directions

- Halve the grapes and set aside.

- Combine the cream cheese, yogurt, sugar and vanilla extract until well mixed.

- Add the grapes into the mixture and pour into a large serving dish

- In a separate dish, combine the brown sugar with the pecans and use this to top the grapes mixture completely.

- Refrigerate for at least an hour, then serve.

Sweet Cherries

Total time: 2 hours, 10 minutes

Cook time: 10 minutes

Refrigerator time: 2 hours

Yield: 4 servings

Ingredients

- ½ kg fresh cherries, washed and pitted
- 2 cups of water
- ¾ cup sugar
- 15 peppercorns
- 1 small vanilla bean, split
- 3 strips orange zest
- 3 strips lemon zest

Directions

- Set cherries aside.

- Add rest of ingredients to a saucepan and bring to a boil, stirring constantly until all the sugar is dissolved.

- Now, add the cherries and simmer for about 10 minutes until soft but not disintegrated.

- Pour out the foam on the surface and set aside to cool.

- Put in the fridge for about 2 hours.

- Strain the liquid before serving.

- Best enjoyed when served with ice cream.

Summer Delight

Total time: 2 hours 10 minutes

Prep time: 2 hour 10 minutes

Cook time: 0 minutes

Yield: 3 servings

Ingredients

- ⅓ kg peaches, sliced

- 2 tbsp. freshly squeezed lemon juice

- ½ bottle of sweet red wine

- 1 tbsp. brown sugar

Directions

- Dip the peach slices in lemon to prevent oxidation.

- Pour the wine in a bowl and add sugar to it, then pour in the peaches together with their juice.

- Cover the bowl and refrigerate for at least 2 hours.

- Serve cold.

Sweetened Roasted Figs

Total time: 1 hour

Prep time: 5 minutes

Cook time: 30 minutes

Refrigerator time: 1 hour

Yield: 4 servings

Ingredients

- 12 ripe figs

- ½ cup sugar

- Ricotta cheese

Directions

- Preheat your oven to 450°F and arrange figs on a baking dish standing upright.

- Meanwhile spread sugar on a skillet and place on low heat.

- Shake the skillet to distribute the sugar when it starts melting.

- Continue doing this until all the sugar melts, about 15 minutes.

- Pour caramel over figs.

- Now roast the figs in the caramel for 15 minutes and set aside to cool.

- Refrigerate the figs for an hour.

- Arrange the figs on plates and drizzle with the caramel.

- Top with the ricotta cheese.

Citrus, Honey and Cinnamon

Total time: 10 minutes

Prep time: 5 minutes

Cook time: 5 minutes

Yield: 4 servings

Ingredients

- 4 oranges

- 2 tbsp. orange flower water

- 2 tbsp. raw honey

- 1 cinnamon stick

- 2 ½ tbsp. toasted and sliced walnuts

Directions

- Peel the oranges and slice them thinly in round shapes.

- Arrange the oranges on a bowl.

- Meanwhile, in a small, heavy saucepan, combine orange flower water, honey and cinnamon stick.

- Stir gently over low heat until the mixture starts simmering, about 2 minutes.

- Pour the hot liquid on the oranges and let it cool, then top with walnuts.

- Best served when cold.

Conclusion

It's common knowledge that people in countries in the Mediterranean region live longer and suffer less, than most people across the globe, from chronic illnesses such as heart diseases, cancer, and type 2 diabetes. The Mediterranean diet is an active lifestyle that involves eating fresh, healthy, and natural ingredients.

Of all the basic tenets in life, health and nutrition rank first. Your first priority should always be to provide your body with quality nutrition—and what better way than the Mediterranean diet?

If you have tried a thousand ways to lose weight without success, this is your best time to start. If you do this, by the same time next week, you will be several pounds lighter, thanks to this amazing diet—and week after week you will be a healthier and lighter version of who you are now.

The tasty recipes in this book will help place healthy food in the heart of your home, and they will help you have great family fun time during meals.

Feel free to tweak the recipes and substitute certain ingredients with your favorite ones to make your very own signature dish.

Again, thank you for buying my book; I hope you enjoyed reading it as much as I enjoyed writing it!

Oh! And one more thing...

...I Need Your Help!

I would love to hear what you thought of my book. I would honestly, wholeheartedly, appreciate it if you left an honest review for me on Amazon.

Thank you and I wish you all the best as you embark on your health journey... May you have great health and motivation as you seek to find health and joy with the help of the Mediterranean diet!

Made in the USA
Middletown, DE
03 November 2016